Hashimotos Thyroiditis Diet and Cookbook

Everything You Need to Know About Hashimotos Disease, Treatments, and Diet Plans to Lead a Productive Life

By Cailin Chase

Disclaimers

Hashimotos Thyroiditis Diet and Cookbook

Table of Contents

Introduction

Hashimoto's thyroiditis is a form of thyroid disease which occurs as a result of a change in your body's immune system. It causes the thyroid to become under-active and, as you are no doubt aware, its symptoms are wide-ranging and often unpleasant. This book is aimed at helping you get through the worst of these symptoms as well as guiding you through the whole process from getting a diagnosis to getting successful treatment with a range of therapies plus special dietary advice and cookbook with lots of delicious and nutritious recipes to look after your thyroid.

We'll focus on the kinds of symptoms you are likely to be experiencing and how you can relay these feelings to your doctor. You will be able to get them to empathise with you and as such they will be able to best understand how they can help you to minimise and overcome as many of the symptoms as possible.

The symptoms of thyroid disease, though known, are notoriously vague in nature. As such, it can be difficult to get a definitive diagnosis in many cases. This is not quite the case with Hashimoto's thyroiditis as it is caused by an alteration in the immune system which can be picked up by a blood test. The problem lies in the fact that other causes of these symptoms and even other causes of thyroid disease are more common. This means that it may take your doctor a while to come to the correct conclusion. With this book in hand, you'll be able to hurry this process along and start getting the treatment you need to start feeling better.

Since thyroid disease is a hormonal condition, it can have wide ranging effects as the multitude of symptoms you are feeling would suggest. We'll also discuss some of the wider implications of living with Hashimoto's thyroiditis, including reproduction and the menopause.

1

Through an explanation of exactly what Hashimoto's thyroiditis is, you'll be able to gain an understanding of the kinds of treatment available from conventional medical sources as well as those alternative therapies increasingly approved of by doctors and patients alike.

One of the major ways by which your symptoms can be alleviated is through dietary change, so this book will outline a food plan for you to follow as well as a list of recipes to help you do so.

What is the thyroid and how does Hashimoto's Thyroiditis affect me?

Hashimoto's thyroiditis is an autoimmune condition which causes the body's immune system to attack itself in error. It results in a loss of function or under-activity of the thyroid gland, known as hypothyroidism. To gain an understanding of what this means, it is necessary to go into a little more detail about what the thyroid's function is in the body.

The thyroid is a small gland which sits at the base of your neck over your windpipe, and is one of several components of your body's endocrine, or hormonal, regulatory system. For such a small gland, it is responsible for a proportionally large number of bodily processes, and this is why its malfunction causes such a wide range of symptoms. It is of particular importance in metabolic and reproductive processes and thus this book aims to provide advice and support about what can be done to minimise the effects of Hashimoto's thyroiditis.

The thyroid, just like other organs and hormonal processes, is controlled in somewhat the same way as a thermostat in your home. When more heat is needed to balance the temperature at home, the thermostat is able to detect this and do something about it. This of course works the other way around too when it is too hot. Ordinarily, the thyroid gland works in the same manner so that your thyroid hormones are produced in the right amounts for your body.

The hormones of the thyroid gland will be discussed in more detail in a later chapter, but for now if is sufficient to say that they have wide-ranging and varied effects on almost all bodily processes, including:

- Metabolism, appetite and body temperature
- Mood and memory
- Cholesterol levels
- Immune system
- Reproductive functions
- Muscles, joints and increased fatigue
- Bone density

In the case of Hashimoto's thyroiditis, the body's immune system undergoes a change which causes it to be unable to properly recognise the thyroid as being one of its own organs. Normally the body produces special proteins known as antibodies to fight against each specific threat it comes across, such as different infections. When the body becomes unable to recognise its own components then auto-antibodies are produced, which are proteins that mistakenly target and attack the body's own cells as if they were foreign invaders. The result is that the thyroid becomes unable to produce hormones in the required amounts.

Another thing is that autoantibodies might be present in many people, yet they never go on to develop any symptoms at all. It isn't always understand why this might be, but it is clear that there are other factors at play in diseases such as Hashimoto's thyroiditis. The ultimate cause of Hashimoto's thyroiditis is unknown but it and other autoimmune diseases do seem to run in families and thus can be said to have a genetic component. But this is by no means the end of the story as there is evidence to suggest that a number of environmental factors have a role to play. These include:

- Diet
    a.   High iodine intake
    b.   Selenium deficiency

c. Vitamin D deficiency

d. Gluten intolerance

- Pollution, including mercury
- Ageing
- Stress
- Imbalances in blood sugar
- Leaky gut
- Infections
- Smoking
- Alcohol consumption

It is perfectly understandable that you would like to know why you are feeling unwell and what can be done about it but as with all thyroid disease, Hashimoto's thyroiditis is more likely to affect simply if you are female, and the unfortunate thing is that it is simply not known why.

Nevertheless, many things can be done to alleviate the symptoms and to allow you to lead a perfectly full life with some adjustments. A great number of different treatment plans and methods have arisen in an effort to combat the effects of this disease. It is important to replace the hormones no longer being produced and the conventional medical treatment focuses on a simplistic replacement of these compounds. While this can often be effective, many people find that it is difficult to find the right dosage for them as individuals, not to mention the fact that your body needs different levels of hormones at different times.

This is where alternative, holistic therapies come into their own. They will be outlined in this book, so that you can choose the kinds of treatment that appeal to you the most. There is even a set of dietary recommendations that have been shown to significantly reduce the effects of the disease and provide a very useful adjunct to medical and holistic therapies. This is completely possible with the right support and the easiest thing to start with is the food you eat, and that's precisely why we are going to focus primarily on dietary change.

Typical Symptoms

The symptoms that occur as a result of under-activity of the thyroid, as is the case in Hashimoto's thyroiditis, are varied and often quite generic in nature. That is to say that they are symptoms which are difficult to define and explain, and thus it can be quite hard to get a definitive diagnosis and treatment plan in place. This can be particularly true as initially the symptoms of Hashimoto's thyroiditis can present as if the thyroid has become overactive. This chapter aims to look at the most common and most debilitating of the symptoms caused by the under-activity of the thyroid in Hashimoto's thyroiditis.

One of the first things you might notice, even before you start feeling ill, is a slight swelling in your neck at the level of the thyroid, that is just below the Adam's apple. This is known as a goitre, and initially it may be small and painless. Eventually though, it may become more tender and swallowing might become irritating or painful as a result. This is one of the first clues of Hashimoto's thyroiditis and your doctor should see it as a call to action, particularly when you tell him all about your other symptoms, some of which are discussed below.

Under-activity of the thyroid generally causes your body as a whole to start to slow down. Your metabolism shuts down so that everything you eat is processed much more slowly by your body, and this makes you prone to weight gain. It becomes harder to maintain a healthy weight even when eating normal amounts of food. This can have a devastating effect on your self-esteem and body image, aside from my health issues.

Everyone wants to feel good about themselves, and with the help of the right treatment and a little extra attention over what you eat and drink, you won't have to worry about this any longer. The dietary plan in this book is aimed specifically at helping you feel the best that you can feel by promoting the most healthful food products and recipes suitable for sufferers of Hashimoto's thyroiditis. Diet is increasingly understood to have a significant effect on the status of your thyroid and by focusing on this a little you can feel like a whole new you.

Another effect of your slower metabolism is that your body finds it harder to generate enough heat. This can leave you feeling chilly on even the hottest of summer days. While you can combat this by wearing more layers of clothing, this isn't really ideal and you no doubt don't want to have to wear winter clothes all through summer. With the help of the advice in this book, you can shed some of those layers and wear whatever you feel best in, without worrying about catching a chill.

Your muscles need a healthy thyroid in order to work properly, and this means that you might have been feeling exhausted most of the time. It's no fun when even a short walk up the street leaves you tired and out of breath. Your muscles might ache and cramp up upon the slight exertion. The same might happen to your joints. All in all, it is not particularly conducive to the kind of life you'd like to lead. With a few tweaks to your diet here and there, and the advice of expert professionals you'll be able to open up a path to a better and more active future.

One of the major things you may well have noticed is that your mood has dropped. As with all chronic diseases, Hashimoto's thyroiditis might easily be confused with depression. The issue lies in separating one from the other. After all, some of the symptoms of thyroid disease don't exactly leave you jumping for joy so you might feel depressed. The problem is that depression in itself, even in the absence of thyroid problems, makes you feel the same way. It may all look a bit chicken-and-egg, so it's important to try to work out which is which.

Commonly, your loss in appetite in thyroid disease does not mean that you lose weight, whereas in depression without thyroid problems your weight is more closely linked with your appetite. This is one way by which you can differentiate the two. Also, thyroid disease means that you'll still feel tired after what would be considered a good night's sleep. Depression as a stand-alone issue would not mean that you were unable to recover from fatigue.

Regardless of the true cause of your low feelings, whether it is due to Hashimoto's thyroiditis itself or the result of how it makes you feel having to live it, the important thing is learning how to help yourself recover from it. When you make the dietary changes that are recommended here, you'll notice that your mood will improve just as your other symptoms will be minimised. You can also talk to your healthcare professionals about ways to help improve your mood.

The majority of thyroid disease sufferers are female, and unfortunately this comes with its own set of problems. Hashimoto's thyroiditis is likely to mean that your menstrual periods have become heavier. Thyroid complaints may also have an effect on fetal development so it is always very important to discuss this with your doctor if you are planning to conceive.

Making a Difficult Diagnosis Easier

One of the most problematic things with thyroid disease as a whole is its diagnosis. This is in part due to the generic and all-encompassing nature of the symptoms. The kinds of things you'll be feeling, such as low mood, anxiety, fatigue and weight gain are often explained away by vague concepts of some kind of inability to deal with the rigors of modern life.

Even if your doctor has the wit to take your symptoms completely seriously, their non-specific nature means that it is entirely possible that they may be thought of as being more to do with medical problems such as:

- Depression and other mood disorders
- Chronic Fatigue Syndrome
- Fibromyalgia
- Anxiety disorders

Naturally, it is intensely frustrating when your problems are just swept aside or misjudged in this manner, and fortunately the medical profession is becoming better at not simply dismissing such so-called generic symptoms. Your doctor is obligated to look for thyroid disease if any of the symptoms discussed earlier are present. The good news is that a diagnosis can be made fairly rapidly once the right tests are conducted.

One of the most difficult aspects of being properly diagnosed so that you can start on getting yourself well again is explaining and describing your symptoms to your doctor so that you can take the thyroid function tests that you need. The best thing to do is to make a list in advance of all the different kinds of things that you are feeling, no matter how irrelevant they may seem. The general nature of many of the symptoms may make this a bit difficult, but the more your doctor knows about how you truly feel from within the easier it will be for you to obtain the correct diagnosis. The more specific you are about each symptom the better.

As was mentioned earlier in this book, your environment and lifestyle play a great role in the kinds of diseases and medical issues that you are susceptible to. If you are still gaining weight even having tried dieting, or if you feel constantly tired despite giving yourself an extra couple of hours of sleep per night, then it's worth mentioning this. Also, let your doctor know if you or anyone around you has noticed differences in your personality.

The fact that autoimmune diseases run in the family means that it is worth telling your doctor about this, as they will then be much more likely to be thinking about the correct diagnosis.

Once you have taken blood tests for thyroid function and thyroid auto-antibodies, if you have Hashimoto's thyroiditis then you'll know about it at this point. Usually the correct kinds of blood tests to do are as follows:

- Thyroid-stimulating hormone (TSH)
- Free thyroxine (T4)
- Free triiodothyronine (T3)
- Autoantibodies
     a.   Anti-thyroid peroxidase (anti-TPO)
     b.   Anti-thyroglobulin (anti-Tg)
     c.   Anti-microsomal

Typically the autoantibodies present can be found in isolation or as a combination. Ultimately, the specific mix is not of much importance in terms of current treatment plans as the end result is the same: the destruction of the thyroid follicles which produce and store T3 and T4. The importance of the presence of the particular types of autoantibodies for treatment purposes may change in the future as medicines to specifically target them are developed.

As mentioned earlier, the initial stages of Hashimoto's thyroiditis may provoke an increase in thyroid function due to inflammation which causes mass release of stored hormones. This is known as thyrotoxicosis and may be a red herring. In time this passes and the symptoms of under-activity described take hold instead.

You can now focus on a treatment plan, taking into account a holistic approach and dietary change as well as conventional medical advice. When you consider your body as the whole entity that it is, you can focus on combating the full range of physical and psychological issues that Hashimoto's thyroiditis has brought up.

Conventional Treatment

The way in which modern medicine attempts to treat thyroid diseases such as Hashimoto's thyroiditis is to simply replace the hormones that are no longer being produced by the body. As many bodily functions rely on thyroid hormones to function optimally, it is very important to maintain a proper level of thyroid hormones in the bloodstream.

The thyroid normally produces two kinds of closely related hormones, known scientifically as thyroxine (T4) and triiodothyronine (T3). You may recognise the former of the two as it is used as a conventional replacement therapy. Generally, only thyroxine is used in conventional treatment because it is far more potent than T3. Most of the effects of the thyroid hormones are believed to be dependent mostly upon thyroxine.

Upon your diagnosis, your doctor will likely suggest that you take thyroxine as part of a replacement therapy. This can be very useful to begin with, but you may find that it is not always easy to find the right dosage for your body. Also, your body's requirements change over time such that what was once a suitable dose may no longer be.

Another major issue of taking pharmaceutical drugs is that they often have undesirable side effects or interactions with other medications. On a similar note, some medicines that you take for other conditions may have an effect on thyroid function, causing, for example, a reduction in T4 production and release. Different types of foods and supplements may also reduce your ability to absorb the T4 found in the medications given to you by your doctor, and you should let them know if you use any of the following:

- Calcium supplements
- Iron supplements
- Multivitamins
- Soy products
- High fiber foods
- Antacids (if they contain aluminum hydroxide)
- Cholestyramine (to lower your cholesterol)
- Sodium polystyrene sulfate (to lower your blood potassium)
- Sucralfate (for ulcers)

With this in mind, a focus on other methods of treatment may be advisable as an adjunct to conventional therapy. There are many factors involved in the development of Hashimoto's thyroiditis and nothing is ever completely set in stone. The conclusion to be drawn from this is that alteration of the presence of reversible environmental causative factors may assist you in ridding yourself of some of the most unpleasant symptoms of thyroid disease.

In addition, treating your body as the whole that it is may be of more benefit than focusing on just the one organ that is affected. Some of the more holistic therapies available may allow your body to return in part to the way it functioned before your thyroid issues. A fundamental concept common to all holistic therapies is the idea that you cannot treat a disease as an individual entity cut off from all other aspects of your body. Thus holistic therapy takes your body as a whole and attempts to make an overall difference, rather than narrow-mindedly focusing on just one aspect of your health and well-being.

Even practitioners of modern medicine are increasingly becoming aware of the benefits of a more holistic approach to healthcare. More and more studies are being conducted that show that some alternative therapies can have a significant and worthwhile effect on your body. You are more likely than ever to be able to discuss your specific issues with your doctor or a range of holistic healthcare practitioners.

This is not to say that modern medicine has no use. On the contrary, the use of thyroxine has been successful in many cases and has been extensively proven to work in clinical studies. Rather, holistic therapies and dietary change can be used as an adjunct to medical treatment to provide that extra bit of help that medication alone cannot provide.

Alternative Therapies

There are an abundance of holistic, alternative therapies that you can try and that many patients have found to be of great help. The most significant change you can make to aid and maintain your recovery is to change your diet, but these holistic methods can be an extremely useful adjunct, particularly when it comes to reducing your stress and anxiety levels and boosting your mood and self-esteem. This is critical, as the better you feel as a person the less your symptoms will bother you even if they are still present.

While it is advisable to continue with conventional medical treatments and to inform your doctor if you intend to participate in any form of other treatment, it is worth investigating different holistic methods in order to find one or more that suit you as an individual. If is often found that conventional medicine is helpful but sometimes cannot quite scratch the itch, so to speak. This is where alternative, holistic therapies come in, as they focus on you as a whole person and unique individual rather than as a collection of organs and tissues to be medicated.

Natural Sources of Thyroid Hormones

While the importance of hormone replacement in treating Hashimoto's thyroiditis cannot be understated, you may not wish not take artificial forms of hormones. Fortunately, if this is indeed the case, there is another option as before modern pharmaceutical drugs were used thyroid conditions were often treated with natural analog. In the beginning, people with thyroid problems were advised to eat animal thyroid organs to obtain the required hormones, but this seems to be a very unpredictable way of ensuring that you get enough at the right times.

Since those times, natural extracts have been developed that don't require you to eat what you may imagine to be something quite unpleasant. Instead, nowadays you can take extracts that have been derived from the hormones found in pig thyroids. Unfortunately however, the problem of variability in hormone quantity has not gone away and such extracts may not provide you with a constant, predictable dose of T4 or T3. Furthermore, each animal species has a different ratio of T4 to T3, meaning that you might not be taking the right amount of each to minimise your symptoms in the way that pharmaceutical-grade thyroxine might.

Exercise

One of the best ways to improve your overall health and mood is to find a form of exercise that you enjoy. It does not have to be particularly vigorous in nature, especially given that you may tire easily. The main thing about exercise is that you are doing something that you enjoy and you are doing it on a regular basis.

Exercise is beneficial on a purely physical level as well as psychologically rewarding. When you work out, even if only gently, your brain releases a set of "feel good" chemicals known as endorphins. The release of these compounds is the reason why many people who exercise enjoy doing it so much.

Perhaps there is a particular sport or activity that you've always enjoyed, or maybe you want to try something new. One such new thing could be yoga, which is becoming increasingly popular all around the world. It is a gentle form of exercise originating in India and is based on specific stretches and slow movements designed to enable you to relax and reduce stress levels at the same time as toning your muscles and improving your breathing. There are several different types of yoga and you can talk with a qualified instructor about your limitations and thus find out the kind of yoga that you would most benefit from.

Often it is easier to get started on an exercise regime if you get a trusted partner to join in. Perhaps your spouse or a close friend would like to take part in your new exercise plan. You might want to invite them have a light-hearted game of tennis or badminton, or perhaps you'd like to have a go at team sports. You'll have a great source of support and can use this newfound activity time to bond further.

Though you'll no doubt be excited to try new things, it is important to also remember your limits. If you exhaust yourself straight away, you may be less likely to continue with your plans and will end up back at square one. Take things gradually and you'll certainly reap the rewards with improved fitness and a better mood.

Herbal Remedies

Before modern society developed, we humans had the knowledge of many natural medicinal herbs and plants at our disposal. Nowadays we tend to use pharmaceutical medication to treat our ailments, but actually the majority of these medicines were first derived from plant sources that our ancestors would have made use of. This is true of many of the most commonly used medications such as aspirin, which was originally derived from willow bark and was mentioned by the great Ancient Greek physician Hippocrates.

Given the pharmaceutical qualities of many herbal supplements, it is always vital to discuss their use with a doctor, particularly if you are taking any prescribed or over-the-counter medications of any kind. Despite the awareness of the potential efficacy of many herbal remedies, there is not always enough empirical evidence to suggest that their use is worthwhile. That said, there are definitely some herbal remedies that have been shown to be of use as adjuncts to conventional treatment in cases of reduced thyroid activity, such as is the case in Hashimoto's thyroiditis.

People with Hashimoto's thyroiditis may find that their adrenal system is not working properly and is not producing cortisol in appropriate quantities. This hormone is responsible for helping your body prepare a response to stressful situations, so without the right amount you may be less able to cope with physical or emotional stressors. Siberian Ginseng could be used to help support the adrenal glands and give you a fighting chance against stress.

To increase the conversion rates of T4 into the more active T3, you can use Indian Ginseng which means that you'll boost the level of thyroid hormone function. This may improve many aspects of the symptoms associated with Hashimoto's thyroiditis, but it is most recognised for its effects on the adrenal glands.

One further example of a good herbal remedy to try out is the schisandra berry, which is known to increase glutathione levels. Glutathione is an anti-oxidant naturally produced by your body and as such it is very useful in the fight against any autoimmune condition. Its production may also be raised by consumption of more protein and selenium-rich foods. This will be discussed later.

Always remember that these herbs should be taken only under the advice of a qualified expert. Although they are considered powerful herbal remedies, they should be used as an adjunct to other therapies and dietary changes rather than as a basis for treatment on their own.

Acupuncture

Acupuncture is a Chinese holistic therapy which involves the insertion of sterilised, fine needles into the skin for the purpose of altering the body's energy flow. It had a philosophical basis in that it focuses on our way of life and the idea of there being a fundamental duality in nature. This is the concept of "yin" and "yang" which represent two opposite aspects of any phenomenon. Generally speaking, rest corresponds to "yin" whereas activity corresponds to "yang". This is used in acupuncture alongside the concept of there being a five element system in nature.

The five elements of nature are represented by Wood and Fire as being more "yang", Water and Metal being more "yin", and Earth being a balance between the two. Each organ as a functional system is considered to be related to each one of these elements and an acupuncturist will assess overall health according to the effects of yin and yang on a person life force.

This natural life force is known as "Qi" and might be considered as our vital life energy. Practitioners of acupuncture believe that Qi and the channels through which it passes in the body are knocked out of balance. It is said to be this imbalance that contributes towards disease states. Though a difficult concept to comprehend for those of us, particularly in the West, and despite the fact that many of us might be skeptical, many people have been treated successfully by qualified acupuncturists for a wide range of diseases.

One of the major benefits of acupuncture and in fact Chinese medical concepts as a whole is the fact that they put the patient first. You are at the center of the diagnostic and treatment process and it is believed that your individuality as a person should inform the specific treatment method that is applied. Additionally, the general aim of acupuncture is to assist your body in reaching a natural equilibrium, otherwise known as homeostasis. This focus on your overall well-being can be helpful and beneficial to you in its own right, regardless of the physical effects it might have.

Aromatherapy and Massage

Essential oils derived from all manner of fragrant plants have been used for thousands of years for their potential effects on illnesses. It has been increasingly shown by empirical scientific evidence that the properties of such oils known to our ancestors are genuine and can be used to effectively treat a range of diseases and symptoms.

Essential oils enter the body via the skin, and when you breathe in they have an effect on your sense of smell and are absorbed by your lungs and hence your bloodstream. Frequently this is accomplished by means of massaging the essential oils mixed with a carrier oil into the skin. Regardless of the medicinal effects of such oils, the act of having a massage in extremely relaxing in itself and may help to relieve some of the stress and anxiety that you have been feeling as a result of Hashimoto's thyroiditis.

The most commonly recommended essential oils for use in treatment of Hashimoto's thyroiditis are:

To improve your concentration and mental clarity:

- Rosemary
- Eucalyptus
- Lemon

To help detoxify your body during weight loss:

- Juniper
- Grapefruit

Of course, aromatherapy is most commonly associated with massage therapies and rightly so, as this is wonderful way to relax and improve your mood, but there are many other ways in which you could incorporate aromatherapy into your life. Oil for the face and hair as well as shower gels and bath oils can be made using the principles of aromatherapy, so that you can enjoy its effects from the comfort of your own home. Essential oils can also be used in room vaporisers and even in your laundry, so that you can feel your favorite scent on your body all day long.

Homeopathy

Homeopathy is based on the idea that any causative substance can also have the opposite effect, a restorative effect. In essence it is the idea that "like cures like". Homeopathic remedies are formulated by diluting an active substance in water until there is almost nothing of the original substance left. This is believed by practitioners of homeopathy to have the effect of magnifying the properties of the original ingredient.

The very concept of homeopathy has been placed under great scrutiny by the medical professional at large, and it is highly unlikely that homeopathy will be recommended as an effective treatment method by your conventional doctor. However, if you feel that it is something that is worth trying out then there are documented cases of any harm being caused as a result of these ideas. Furthermore, not all effects on disease are physical in nature and you may benefit in other ways that have a knock-on effect on your physical health.

Laser therapy

It's worth noting that some clinical trials have been done in the past few years that have suggested that low level laser therapy involving near-infrared light may have a beneficial effect on autoimmune-mediated thyroid diseases. As this is a recent development, this is not something that you can pursue as a treatment method at this time, but it may well be something to think about in the future.

Diet

Given the large number of potential dietary factors involved in the development of Hashimoto's thyroiditis, it makes a lot of sense to alter your diet in order to reduce your symptoms to a minimum. There are various dietary protocols that have been extensively researched in terms of autoimmune disease as a whole, and they have been shown to be effective in relation to Hashimoto's thyroiditis as well. This kind of a diet and overview of its rules, with some added things specific to Hashimoto's thyroiditis, will be demonstrated through a collection of recipes at the end of this book.

One of the most common reasons for the development of Hashimoto's thyroiditis is gluten intolerance. There are similarities between one of the parts of the gluten molecule, known as gliadin, and proteins in the thyroid gland. This means that if you are gluten intolerant then consumption of gluten may result in your immune system producing antibodies that attack the thyroid gland as well as targeting the gliadin molecule. If there is any chance that you might be intolerant to gluten, it is best to avoid it completely and the diet included in this book will show you how.

If you do choose to consume carbohydrates then you should not only ensure that they do not contain gluten but also that they are complex in nature. The consumption of gluten-free will allow you to digest carbohydrates and release their energy slowly, thus avoiding the insulin spike that leads to quick energy bursts and then burnout and fatigue.

Ordinarily, insulin is secreted by the pancreas to allow the cells in your body to take in glucose, or blood sugar. High or low blood sugar as a result of the wrong kind of diet can impact the thyroid gland, causing its destruction and thus a reduction in thyroid hormones in the bloodstream. The consumption of too many carbohydrates over time causes the cells in the body to become too used to the presence of glucose in the blood and as such they start to become resistant to its effects. The repeated insulin spikes caused by a high carbohydrate diet eventually cause type 2 diabetes and other complications. This is a vicious cycle that could affect your thyroid even more so it is vitally important that carbohydrate consumption is kept under control, particularly the consumption of simple processed sugars as found in candy and cakes.

On the flip side of this, low blood sugar can also negatively affect the thyroid over time. The body considers a lack of blood sugar to be an stressor and as such your adrenal glands will produce more cortisol, the chronic stress hormone. Cortisol is actually useful to the body in the right concentration, in this case to cause the liver to release some stored glucose and bring blood levels so up to normal. However, in the case of frequent low blood sugar cortisol is released in a manner that causes the pituitary gland, a kind of hormonal control switch in the brain, to function at a lower rate. This means that the thyroid is not stimulated by the thyroid-stimulating hormone released by the pituitary gland and thus does not release as much T4 and T3 as is required.

Dietary fiber should also be consumed to improve but health and thus aid weight loss and a reduction in any digestive symptoms you may have. Though our guts themselves cannot digest many forms of such fiber, the bacteria naturally present in our intestines thrive on such things. The best sources of fiber are fruits and vegetables, and they should be forming the majority of your diet. Furthermore, the kinds of gut bacteria that use fiber as fuel have been shown to have a positive effect on your cholesterol levels, reducing the low density lipoprotein cholesterol (LDL), the so-called "bad" cholesterol.

Everyone knows that our bodies require special substances known as vitamins in order to function properly. Without a proper supply of these vitamins, autoimmune conditions such as Hashimoto's thyroiditis can be caused and made worse.

One vitamin of great importance is vitamin D, which we primarily derive from our skin in response to exposure to sunlight. Nowadays, as we spend more and more time indoors, it can be difficult for our bodies to make as much vitamin D as we need.

Without vitamin D, our immune systems are much less well regulated and disease states can result, in particular autoimmune thyroid diseases such as Hashimoto's thyroiditis.

Unfortunately, it is not so simple to fix as getting more exposure to sunlight or eating vitamin D-enriched foods. The reason for this is several fold. Dietary forms of vitamin D are absorbed in the small intestine and, as is common in Hashimoto's thyroiditis, any inflammation in this area of our bowels can reduce our ability to absorb certain vitamins.

In addition, vitamin D is fat-soluble which means we need to eat enough fat in order to absorb such vitamins. This can be hard to do while trying to lose weight due to dietary restrictions, so it is important to consume a healthy source of fats such as olive oil. Furthermore, fats and oils contain essential fatty acids which our bodies cannot produce themselves and must source them from our diets. These fatty acids are vital for the growth of skin, hair and nails, so the inclusion of good sources of healthy fats and oils in your diet may help any symptoms of hair thinning that you may have.

Vitamin B12 contributes to many bodily functions and an increase in consumption of products containing vitamin B12 may help to combat fatigue and tiredness. It is most commonly found in abundance in animal products, and as such vegetarians may find themselves lacking.

One of the most common mineral deficiencies associated with thyroid disease is a lack of selenium. This is a trace metal found in many foods in small doses but it can be difficult to get as much of it as the body needs. Without selenium, our immune systems cannot work at their optimum level and as such we put ourselves at risk of increased likelihood of infections and autoimmune diseases. One of the best ways to increase selenium intake is to consume a few Brazil nuts every day as they are especially rich in this important mineral.

To sum up all of this wealth of dietary information and advice, most people find that they benefit from adhering to a dietary regime that cuts out gluten-containing grains and focuses on the consumption of fruits and vegetables alongside healthful lean meats. It is important to maintain a balanced diet in this manner, making sure that portion size is under control. Additionally, caffeine and alcohol ought to be avoided for the most part.

The remainder of this book focuses on providing a number of recipes for you to use to ensure that you keep your symptoms to a minimum and start to feel a whole new you.

Cookbook

The autoimmune protocol, which is advised to be followed by everyone who suffers from autoimmune disorders, follows all the principles discussed in the previous chapter. It is based on a diet that is directed at minimising inflammation and reducing the overstimulation of the immune system. While autoimmune conditions do not necessarily vanish, their symptoms can be reduced significantly if you follow these principles.

As mentioned previously, autoimmune diseases share some of the same mechanisms of action in the body, but each kind of disease has its own specific features too. Furthermore, we all differ from person to person so some things will work better for some people rather than others, but it is hoped that everyone will find something that is helpful to them.

Generally speaking, for the recovery of your immune system it is best to avoid grains as they often contain gluten. Legumes, that is to say beans, should also be removed from your diet as they contain anti-nutrients which will prevent your gut from absorbing the kinds of nutrients that you need to recover your health. All products containing alcohol and added sugar should be eliminated as they are not really useful to your body and are essentially empty calories, not to mention the fact that they have an overall inflammatory effect in your gut and may thus further exacerbate your thyroid problems. You can, however, eat green beans and string beans as they do not contain the same kinds of anti-nutrients as other beans.

While the majority of fruits and vegetables are strongly encouraged and will certainly help you to fix your immune system and gain relief from the symptoms of Hashimoto's thyroiditis, there are some that ought to be avoided. Plants from the nightshade family should particularly avoided as they are known to cause gastrointestinal discomfort and have a generally inflammatory influence on the body. Such plants to be avoided include tomatoes, white potatoes, onions, bell peppers and chilli peppers, and aubergines.

Though usually great source of protein, eggs should really be avoided if you have an autoimmune complaint like Hashimoto's thyroiditis. This is because some of the protein components of the egg-white can pass through the gut lining intact, which means that the cells of the immune system can be stimulated, resulting in an exacerbation of your symptoms.

It is best to get your protein from quality, organic grass-fed animal products and wild-caught fish wherever possible to ensure that you are not consuming any unwanted chemicals such as nitrates which are commonly used to preserve meat products. Processed meat products such as pre-packaged bacon may be irritant to your gut as a result of their nitrate content.

Dairy products such as milk, cheese and yogurt should not be consumed if you are suffering from any autoimmune condition. This is partly due to the fact that many of us are lactose-intolerant, often without even realising it. As such, the attempt to digest lactose may cause irritation and damage to the gut. As mentioned before, damage to the gut may result in further damage to the thyroid which is what you definitely don't want. A useful and nutritious substitute that can be used in many recipes is coconut milk.

Fermented products are generally good for your gut flora, helping to promote the growth of bacteria which are beneficial to your digestive system. While you ought not to consume any fermented dairy products or soy products, there are alternative ways in which to get the same effects to benefit your immune system. Some of the most delicious ways to enjoy fermented foods and drinks are in the form of sauerkraut, kimchi and kombucha.

In general, nuts and seeds ought to be avoided, as well as their oils, as they are high in the same kinds of anti-nutrients as grains and legumes. They also tend to have an inflammatory effect on the body. The only exception that you may wish to make is for Brazil nuts, if you are able to tolerate them and they do not cause your symptoms to flare up, as they contain high levels of selenium which is very useful for combatting Hashimoto's thyroiditis. Alternatively, you could take a selenium supplement if recommended by a healthcare professional.

As fats are an important part of your diet and are vital in the production of healthy skin, hair and nails it is crucial that you find a good source of healthy fats that you enjoy on a daily basis. Most commonly, this is olive oil but you could also consider using coconut oil or animal fats in moderation. As mentioned above, seed oils should be avoided.

Further to the effects of aberrations in blood sugar levels on the thyroid and your overall health, it is recommended that you limit fruit intake to one or two portions per day. This is also important as a kind of fruit sugar, fructose, common to all fruits can have an irritant effect on your gastrointestinal tract if consumed in excess. By keeping your gut healthy, you'll be contributing to your thyroid health as well as your general well-being.

All of these different dietary alternations and outright bans must seem very restrictive at first glance, and such an assumption is absolutely understandable. However, there are many things that you still can eat, as well as many innovative alterations that can be made so that you can enjoy analogs of your favourite foods and recipes. At the very least, you could try adopting this way of eating for a month and see if you feel the benefit. Many people give it a try and they go on to continue with this way of eating for years and often forever.

You can always slowly reintroduce some food groups over time to see which specific things your body is most sensitive to. You can then make an informed decision about which foods are best for you as an individual. Whatever you decide to do, you now have the power of knowledge and can take the steps forward that you think you need to take.

In reintroducing any food group, care should be taken and the following points should be taken into account:

- Introduce one food at a time to pinpoint each causative food
- Identify any symptoms you notice
- Start with foods that are less likely to cause symptoms:

Egg yolks

1. Seeds and nuts
2. Grass-fed butter
3. Coffee
4. Vegetables (individually)

- Do it slowly (it can take several days for the body to mount a full antibody response to a reintroduced food)
- Do not be afraid to go back to restricting any given food

You will find below a collection of recipes for breakfast, lunch and dinner, plus some snack and drink ideas.

Breakfast

Pumpkin Porridge

1 medium pumpkin, halved

1 cup chilled coconut milk

1 cup strawberries, chopped

2 tbsp shredded coconut, toasted

Cinnamon

1) Preheat the oven to 350 degrees F.

2) Place the pumpkin halves cut side down on a greased, rimmed baking tray. Bake for about 1 hour or until tender and cooked through.

3) When the pumpkin is cool enough to touch, scoop out the seeds and discard them. Scoop out the pumpkin flesh and mash to your desired consistency.

4) Pour the milk over each bowl of pumpkin and add the strawberries, coconut and a sprinkle of cinnamon.

Granola

2 cups coconut flakes

1 tbsp coconut oil

1 1/2 tbsp coconut manna

Zest of 1 orange

1/2 tsp cinnamon

1) Heat coconut oil and coconut manna until the mixture become a pourable liquid.

2) Add cinnamon, stir and remove the mixture from the heat.

3) Add the coconut flakes to a bowl and pour the coconut oil mixture over it. Mix it together gently.

4) Add the orange zest over the mixture.

5) Line a baking tray with baking parchment and pour the coconut mixture and spread it out evenly.

6) Cook in a pre-heated oven at 350 degrees F for 12-15 minutes. Stir the mixture every few minutes to prevent burning of the mixture.

7) Remove from the oven and let cool. Store in an airtight container or consume immediately.

Breakfast Burgers

1 lb ground pork
1 tsp sea salt
1 tsp dried sage
1 tsp dried thyme
1/2 tsp ground ginger
1/2 tsp dried rosemary

1) Place the pork in a large bowl and add the salt, sage, thyme, ginger and rosemary. Mix well.

2) Separate out the mixture into 4 x 4 oz portions and mold each portion into the shape of a burger patty.

3) Put each patty on a flat board and freeze until just firm to the touch. Remove the frozen patties from the board and store the ones that you don't want to cook yet.

4) Cook the patties in a frying pan over a medium heat and until brown on both sides and fully cooked.

5) Serve alongside sauerkraut.

Lunch

Watercress, Beetroot and Orange Salad (serves 3-4)

1 lb raw beetroot, tops removed

3 large oranges

1 tsp white wine vinegar

4 oz watercress

1) Preheat the oven to 375 degrees F.

2) Bake the beetroot covered in foil for 1 hour, until soft.

3) Peel 2 oranges and chop into segments, removing the pith. Collect the juice of the third orange in a bowl.

4) Add the vinegar and oil to the orange juice and combine well. Season to taste.

5) Allow the beetroot to cool slightly before chopping it into chunks.

6) Combine the beetroot, orange segments and watercress. Drizzle the dressing over the salad and serve.

Turkey with Avocado and Grapefruit Relish (serves 2)

For the turkey:

2 turkey breast cuts (approx. 8 oz)

1 tbsp olive oil

Pinch of salt

For the relish:

1 large grapefruit, peeled and cut into segments

1/2 small avocado, peeled and diced

1 tbsp cilantro leaves, chopped

1 tsp red wine vinegar (or cider vinegar)

1) Add the grapefruit segments to a bowl, along with the avocado, cilantro and vinegar. Mix well.

2) Prepare the turkey by lightly salting it.

3) Heat the oil to a medium-high heat in a pan. Add the turkey and cook for 2-3 minutes on each side, so that it is cooked thoroughly.

4) Serve the turkey with the relish and a side of vegetables.

Pâté with Celery, Carrot and Cucumber

1 1/2 lb chicken liver, trimmed and cut into chunks

1 tsp dried sage

1 tsp dried rosemary

1 tsp dried thyme

1 bay leaf

Sea salt

3 tbsp coconut cream

½ cup of coconut oil

1) Melt 2 tbsp of the coconut oil in a frying pan. Add the sage, rosemary, thyme and bayleaf and continue cooking for about 10 minutes.

2) Add the liver to the pan and cook, stirring until it is just cooked through.

3) Transfer the liver to a food processor. Add the coconut milk and remaining ingredients. Blend until smooth.

4) Pour into a serving dish and refrigerate until cold.

5) Serve with slices of cucumber and carrots and celery sticks.

Dinner

Lemon and Thyme Chicken with Rocket Salad (serves 1)

1 skinless chicken breast

1 sprig of thyme

2 tsp olive oil

Juice of 1/2 lemon

Pinch of sea salt and black pepper

For the salad:

3 1/2 oz rocket leaves

1 tbsp extra-virgin olive oil

Pinch of sea salt and black pepper

1) Score the chicken breast on one side with a knife.

2) In a small bowl, mix together the thyme and 1 tsp of the olive oil. Cover the chicken in this mixture.

3) Add the chicken breast to a pan on medium heat, cooking it in the remainder of the olive oil until golden brown.

4) Season with salt, pepper and lemon juice.

5) Combine the salad ingredients in a bowl.

6) Serve the chicken alongside the salad.

Cauliflower Ratatouille (serves 2)

5 1/2 oz cauliflower florets

2 oz zucchini, chopped

1 tbsp thyme leaves

1 tbsp rosemary leaves

Olive oil

Pinch of salt and black pepper

Chopped parsley

1) Preheat the oven to 400 degrees F.

2) Blanch the cauliflower in a saucepan of boiling water. Drain, rinse in cold water and pat dry.

3) Place the vegetables on a baking tray and drizzle with olive oil.

4) Add the chopped thyme and rosemary, and season with salt and pepper.

5) Roast the vegetables for 15-20 minutes until golden brown. Turn them halfway through.

6) Serve with freshly chopped parsley to garnish.

Grilled Trout and Radish Slaw (Serves 4)

4 trout fillets (approx. 1 1/2 lb in total)
1 tbsp olive oil
Pinch of salt and black pepper

For the slaw:
1 cup radish, grated or thinly sliced
1 tbsp parsley, chopped
2 tsp cider vinegar
1/4 tsp ginger, minced
Pinch of salt and black pepper

1) To make the slaw, combine the radish, parsley, vinegar, salt and pepper.

2) Brush the olive oil over the trout fillets and sprinkle them with salt and pepper to taste.

3) Place the fillets skin side down on a grill pan. Grill them for 8-10 minutes, until the flesh flakes easily.

4) Serve the fish with the slaw and a side of sautéed spinach.

Snacks and Drinks

Pickled Gherkins

25 small cucumbers

1/2 lb salt

2 quarts water

0.6 quarts white vinegar

1 tbsp pickling spice

1) Add the salt to the water to make brine.

2) Cover the cucumbers with the brine in a large pan.

3) Heat the liquid to near boiling point, but do not actually boil. Simmer for 10 minutes.

4) Drain the cucumbers and allow to cool.

5) Place the vinegar and pickling spice in a saucepan and bring to the boil for 1 minute.

6) Pack the cucumbers into a warm Kilner jar, and cover with the vinegar.

7) These pickles can be stored for weeks and eaten as a snack whenever you like.

Gingered Carrots

12 oz carrots, peeled and cut into thin strips

2 tbsp olive oil

1 inch ginger root, peeled and grated

Ground black pepper

1) Place the carrots in a bowl and mix in the olive oil and ginger.

2) Cover with cling film and allow the flavors to develop for at least 30 minutes.

3) Season the carrots with black pepper.

4) They can be easily stored and can be eaten any time.

Aloe Vera Smoothie

1/4 cup fresh aloe vera, chopped

1/2 medium cucumber, chopped

1/2 medium banana, chopped

1/2 cup coconut milk (or other milk/milk replacement)

1/2 cup water

Detox Cleansing Smoothie

1/2 cup kale, shredded

1/2 cup mango, cubed

1 medium celery stalk, chopped

1/2 cup oranges, peeled and chopped

2 tbsp fresh parsley, finely chopped

2 tbsp fresh mint, finely chopped

Spinach and Apple Juice

3 1/2 oz baby spinach, shredded

2 oz kale, shredded

1 1/4 oz broccoli

1 small cucumber, halved lengthways

5 oz celery

2 apples, cored and sliced into quarters

3/4 inch root ginger, peeled

1 small handful mint, shredded

1/2 small lemon, peeled and sliced into quarters

1 lime, peeled and sliced into quarters

Conclusion

Thank you for reading this full book. I have written all the information about 'Hashimotos Thyroiditis'. Don't be frustrated about Hashimotos. Knowledge can go a long way in treatment and prevention.

www.ingramcontent.com/pod-product-compliance
Lightning Source LLC
Chambersburg PA
CBHW070829290526
45795CB00002B/885